THE GLUCOSE REVOLUTION METHOD

How Maintaining a Healthy Blood Sugar Level Can Completely Transform Your Life.

Willow Monroe

DISCLAIMER

Every effort has made this book as complete and accurate as possible. This book provides information only up to the publishing date. Therefore, this book should be used as a guide, not the ultimate source.

The purpose of this book is to educate. The author and the publisher do not warrant that the information contained in this book is fully complete and shall not be responsible for any errors or omissions. The author and publisher shall have neither liability nor responsibility to any person or entity concerning any loss or damage caused or alleged to be caused directly or indirectly by this book.

Table Of Content

Introduction

Our blood glucose is a crucial component of our health that is often disregarded despite the significant role it plays in determining our overall wellbeing. This is the narrative of a trip, a change, and a revolution, and it is told through the lens of "The Glucose Revolution Method."

In the area of health, gaining an awareness of the intricacies of blood glucose regulation is analogous to discovering the keys to a life that is full of vitality and energy. A apparently little molecule, blood sugar really has an extraordinary amount of influence on both our physical and mental health. It is the source of the energy that powers every action, every thought, and every beating of our hearts.

However, it is also a power that, if not properly handled, has the potential to disturb our lives and throw a shadow over our health. We, as the keepers of our wellbeing, are the ones who have the secret to managing this precarious equilibrium. You may recover that power by following the instructions in this book.

This is not just another book; rather, it is a guarantee of results. A guarantee that you will be provided with the information and techniques that will enable you to take charge of your health, to realize the transforming potential of the changes you make to your food and lifestyle, and to set off on a path toward regaining your energy and vigor.

Throughout this trip, you will investigate the intriguing science that supports blood sugar management and examine the deep significance of maintaining proper control of your blood sugar levels. You are going to get an understanding of how apparently innocuous food decisions may really have a massive effect on your health and well-being. You are going to learn about the fascinating realm of the glycemic index, which is the key to unlocking the mysteries of maintaining stable blood sugar levels.

However, the content of this book is not limited to theoretical considerations; rather, it focuses on application. We will walk you through the process of developing your very own Glucose-Friendly Diet, assisting you in selecting the appropriate carbs, helping you maintain portion control, and guiding you in the preparation of delectable meals that are also conducive to the achievement of your wellness objectives.

The trip does not come to a conclusion with carbs. As part of your efforts to maintain stable blood sugar, you will investigate the function of fats and proteins. We are going to teach you how to embrace physical exercise as a strong weapon in your armory, which will help you enhance your insulin sensitivity and maintain consistent levels of blood glucose.

Your trip would not be complete without the vital component of consistent monitoring. We will teach you how to interpret the numbers on your blood glucose monitor so that you can make educated choices regarding your food and lifestyle, putting you squarely in control of your own health.

But this revolution isn't only for those who have diabetes; it's for everybody who wants to live a life that's filled to the brim with energy and vitality. In this lesson, we will dig into the area of prevention and give ideas on how to protect against type 2 diabetes and manage blood glucose in a variety of living circumstances.

You will not be on your own to complete this task. We are going to talk about how important it is to surround yourself with a strong support system, make connections with others who work in the medical field, and get involved in groups that have the same objectives as you.

Your adventure starts from this point on. The Glucose Revolution Method is intended to serve as your road map, compass, and guide. It is a promise of change, of taking charge of one's life, and, most importantly, of embracing a life that is full of health and vitality.

I would be honored to welcome you to your glucose revolution.

Chapter 1

Mastering the Glycemic Index

The Glycemic Index (GI) is a concept that is commonly discussed in the field of health and nutrition, although it is usually misinterpreted by those who discuss it. It is like having the key to unlocking greater management of blood sugar, a notion that has the potential to profoundly influence the nutritional decisions we make on a daily basis. In this chapter, we will unlock this code for you, making it completely understandable and applicable in real-world situations.

What is the Glycemic Index?

The Glycemic Index is a numerical scale that classifies carbohydrates in meals depending on how they affect one's blood sugar levels. The lower the number, the less of an impact the carbohydrate has. On this scale, a value is given to each meal that contains carbohydrates. The values on this scale normally range from 0 to 100. The higher the GI value of a meal, the more quickly and significantly it causes the level of glucose in the blood to increase.

To put it more simply, meals that have a high GI are quickly digested and absorbed, which causes fast increases in the amount of sugar in the blood. Foods that have a low GI, on the other hand, take longer to digest and are absorbed even more slowly, which leads to an increase in blood sugar that is more gradual and consistent. The key is not to cut carbs out of your diet entirely but rather to choose your carbohydrate sources carefully.

The Practical Aspect

Let's move on to the practical side now. What does this entail for you in your day-to-day activities? Imagine that you're getting ready to start your day and you have some bread and jam for breakfast. Both the bread and the sweet jam have a high glycemic index (GI). What takes place? Your glucose levels in the blood increase. You could have an initial surge of energy, but it will shortly be followed by a crash that will leave you feeling exhausted and with a yearning for more sweets.

Imagine, instead, a bowl of whole-grain oats topped with a selection of fresh berries as your morning meal. Both the oats and the berries have a relatively low glycemic index. As your blood sugar progressively increases, you get a consistent supply of energy, which enables you to remain attentive and satisfied throughout the process. This is the power that comes from having knowledge of and making use of the glycemic index.

Low-GI vs. High-GI Foods

To become an expert on the Glycemic Index, one of the most important things you need to do is familiarize yourself with the distinctions between meals that have a low GI and those that have a high GI. It's possible that the choices you make about these meals will have a substantial effect not only on your capacity to control your blood sugar levels, but also on your overall health and wellbeing.

High-GI Foods

Many times, refined and processed ingredients are used in the production of foods that have a high glycemic index. They consist of items such as white bread, cereals that are rich in sugar, and the vast majority of snack foods that are processed in some way. Your blood sugar levels will spike after eating meals with a high glycemic index (GI), which will cause you to have an initial burst of energy followed by a dip in your energy levels. Consuming meals with these ingredients will not assist you in reaching your objective of keeping stable blood sugar levels.

Low-GI Foods

Foods with a low glycemic index, on the other hand, are those that are more complex and less processed. These include foods such as legumes, whole grains, and the majority of vegetables and fruits. They are digested slowly, which results in a steady flow of energy over a longer period of time. Consuming meals with a low glycemic index will help you keep your blood sugar levels steady and stave off hunger longer.

But here's the beauty of it: putting meals into high GI or low GI categories is not the only way to think about it. A meal's GI may be affected by a wide variety of variables, including the technique of cooking and the food combinations used. For instance, a baked potato has a high GI, but the overall effect on blood sugar may be mitigated if it is consumed together with a supply of healthy fat and some protein. This is because healthy fat and protein help to keep blood sugar levels stable.

The Science Behind GI and Blood Sugar

Let's go a bit further into the science that behind the Glycemic Index and its influence on blood sugar levels.

Digestion and Blood Sugar

When you eat carbs, your body converts those carbohydrates into glucose, which then gets distributed throughout your body via the bloodstream. These glucose molecules are the principal source of fuel for the cells in your body. The glycemic index (GI) of a diet may have a significant impact on the pace at which carbs are digested and glucose is released into the system.

meals with a high glycemic index induce a fast rise in blood sugar levels because they are rapidly broken down and absorbed, while meals with a low glycemic index cause a rise in blood sugar levels that is gradual and more under control. Those who struggle with diabetes or who want to have a consistent energy level throughout the day are significantly impacted by the significance of these findings.

Hormones and Hunger

To fully appreciate the science that behind the Glycemic Index, one must also comprehend the function of hormones in controlling both blood sugar levels and feelings of hunger. Foods with a high glycemic index (GI) may cause an increase in insulin, which is the hormone that is responsible for bringing blood sugar levels down. However, this sudden drop in blood sugar may bring on feelings of hunger as well as cravings, which can lead to eating more than necessary.

On the other hand, eating meals with a low glycemic index causes an insulin response that is more slow and mild, which helps to control feelings of hunger. This is especially crucial for maintaining a healthy weight as well as for general health.

The Glycemic Load

Even while the Glycemic Index is a helpful tool, it does not provide all of the information. The Glycemic Index (GI) is an extension of the GI that takes into consideration the amount of carbohydrates present in a portion of food. This quantity is referred to as the Glycemic Load (GL). Because it takes into account both the quality and quantity of the carbs in a diet, it offers a more realistic picture of how a food will effect the amount of sugar in the blood.

For instance, watermelon has a high GI, but its GL is relatively modest due to the fact that it only contains a little amount of carbs in each meal. When determining the effect that a meal has on blood sugar, it is essential to take into account both the surrounding circumstances and the quantity of the item consumed.

To sum everything up

As we continue on our journey through The Glucose Revolution Method, we equip ourselves with a potent instrument known as the Glycemic Index. It's not just about the statistics; it's also about the decisions you make and the effects they have. By deciphering this index, you will be able to make more educated choices regarding your food, maintain better control over your blood sugar levels, and, as a result, improve your overall health and vigor.

In the chapters that follow, we will discuss how to design a diet that is friendly to glucose, how to become an expert in the art of selecting the appropriate carbs, and how to comprehend the roles that proteins and fats play in the regulation of blood sugar levels. In addition to this, we are going to go into the topics of the advantages of engaging in regular physical exercise, the relevance of monitoring your glucose levels, and the tactics for avoiding diabetes and having a life that is full of vitality.

On your voyage toward self-improvement, the Glycemic Index will serve as your navigator, your ally, and your compass. Let us seize the power that comes with knowledge, take responsibility for our own health, and prepare for the real revolution that is on the horizon.

Chapter 2

Crafting Your Glucose-Friendly Diet

In the area of blood glucose management, the formulation of a diet that serves as a potent ally in the upkeep of stable and healthy blood sugar levels is the fundamental component of a successful path toward managing blood glucose levels. This chapter acts as a compass for you, guiding you through the complexities of designing a glucose-friendly diet that is beneficial to your health and well-being and supports your goals.

Choosing the Right Carbohydrates

Carbohydrates make up the bulk of our diet, and the decisions we make about this macronutrient group have a significant impact on how much glucose is circulating in our blood. Realizing that not all carbohydrates are created equal is one of the most important steps we can take toward achieving our goal. It's not about cutting off carbohydrates entirely but about making decisions based on the information you have.

Enter the idea of the Glycemic Index, or GI for short, which is an important tool for determining how different types of carbs affect blood sugar. Carbohydrates with a low glycemic index (GI), such whole grains, legumes, and certain fruits and vegetables, are digested more slowly, which results in a more gradual increase in blood sugar levels. On the other hand, carbohydrates with a high glycemic index (GI), such as sweet snacks or refined grains, cause fast rises in blood glucose.

The difficult part is figuring out how to maximize the consumption of low-GI carbs while decreasing the consumption of high-GI foods. It is not about deprivation, but rather about choosing choices that are more sustainable and beneficial to one's health. In this lesson, we are going to go over some useful techniques and suggestions for daily life that will enable you to load your plate with the appropriate carbs, therefore laying a strong basis for your diet that is favorable toward glucose.

Portion Control and Balancing Macronutrients

The notion of controlling portions and maintaining a healthy balance of macronutrients is just as important for us as we continue on our dietetic path. It's not just about the food you eat; the quantity of food you take in is as important. Blood sugar levels are strongly influenced by the sizes of portions consumed. A healthy intake of nutrients may be maintained while preventing unneeded rises in blood glucose if one is aware of and makes an effort to practice proper portion management.

Furthermore, it is essential to strike a healthy equilibrium between the three types of macronutrients, which are proteins, fats, and carbs. This equilibrium optimizes the way in which your body reacts to meals, which in turn contributes to more stable blood sugar levels. We will investigate the science behind this balance and provide you with the knowledge and skills necessary to successfully traverse the world of macronutrients and understand the part they play in a diet that is favorable to glucose.

Planning Glucose-Friendly Meals

The creation of a meal that is glucose-friendly is an art form a beautiful symphony of tastes, nourishment, and the maintenance of stable blood sugar levels. In this part of the document, the theory will be put into practice. We will assist you in formulating meal plans that are not only delectable but also carefully crafted to contribute to the achievement of your fitness objectives.

You will find recipes, meal plans, and practical ways for preparing meals that are geared specifically at maintaining consistent blood sugar levels. You will learn how to construct meals that delight your taste senses while also nourishing your health, and you will learn how to do this for everything from breakfast to supper, from snacks to special occasions.

Participate with us in the investigation of the creation of a diet that is glucose-friendly. Acquire the skills necessary to empower yourself with information, master the art of controlling your portion sizes, and dive into the realm of meal planning in order to create meals that not only benefit your health but also please your taste buds. It is time to turn your diet into a strong asset in your road toward stable blood sugar and overall well-being, and it all starts with making some changes to your diet.

Chapter 3

Foods for Stable Blood Sugar

The meals that we choose to provide sustenance for our bodies are an important thread in the larger tapestry of health. What we take in is more than simply fuel; it's the very core of what it means to live. In addition, the decisions we make may have a significant impact on the degree to which we are able to regulate our blood sugar levels.

In this chapter, we are going to begin our trip into the core of a diet that is favorable toward glucose. We are going to investigate the idea of the Glycemic Index (GI), and then we are going to unveil the mysteries of a low-GI pantry, which is where the magic of maintaining stable blood sugar levels starts.

The Low-GI Pantry

Imagine that your kitchen is a research facility, and that the shelves of your pantry are stocked with products that either help or hinder your blood sugar levels. Let's get down to business and fill this laboratory with expertise and accuracy.

The Glycemic Index is a numerical scale that classifies meals that include carbohydrates based on how rapidly they elevate blood sugar levels. The higher an item is on the Glycemic Index, the more quickly it will rise blood sugar levels. Foods that have a low GI take longer to digest, which results in a rise in blood sugar that is more gradual and consistent. On the other hand, meals with a high glycemic index lead to fast increases and drops in blood sugar.

Barley, quinoa, and steel-cut oats are examples of whole grains that belong in a low-GI pantry. These grains are excellent sources of sustained energy since they do not cause blood sugar levels to fluctuate as much as high-GI foods do. Make the switch from refined flours to whole wheat flour, and choose brown rice over white rice. When you're trying to keep your blood sugar steady, legumes like lentils and chickpeas are your best friends since they're filled with protein. These vital foods not only provide your body the fuel it needs but also supply it with the fiber, vitamins, and minerals it requires.

The pantry also contains nuts, seeds, and the butters made from them; these items provide not just beneficial fats but also an abundance of nutrients. Spices and herbs, which not only contribute to the overall taste of the food you prepare but also have the capacity to regulate blood sugar levels, should not be forgotten either. For example, cinnamon has been investigated for its potential to increase insulin sensitivity and has shown promising results.

Incorporating Whole Grains and Fiber

Whole grains are not only an important component of a low-GI pantry, but they are also the dietary cornerstone of a diet that is favorable to glucose. Blood sugar rises may be naturally mitigated by the presence of fiber in the complex carbs that these foods have in abundance. But they aren't the only advantages you get.

Because fiber contributes to the sensation of fullness, it makes it more difficult to succumb to the urge to overeat and, as a result, assists with portion control, which is an essential component of effective blood sugar management. In addition to this, it promotes the health of the digestive tract, which in turn may help to regulate blood sugar levels.

But how can you ensure that eating healthy grains on a regular basis doesn't seem like a chore? When it comes to your choices of bread, pasta, and cereal, choose for those that include whole grains rather than processed grains. Try your hand at making delicacies such as quinoa salads, barley soups, and pasta made with whole wheat. Both your tongue's tastebuds and your blood sugar will be grateful to you if you do this.

Power of Fruits and Vegetables

A diet low in glucose is associated with brightly colored produce, such as fruits and vegetables, since these foods are low in glucose. They are chock-full of essential nutrients, such as vitamins, minerals, anti-oxidants, and fiber, and might be compared to a natural pharmacy.

When you grab for a piece of fruit or a portion of vegetables, you are not only treating yourself to a delectable and all-natural snack; you are also giving your body the resources it needs to maintain stable blood sugar levels. On average, fruits and vegetables, especially those that are low in starch content, have a low glycemic index.

Berries, for example, are not only delicious and tasty, but they are also densely packed with antioxidants, which may help to boost general health. The nutritious density of leafy greens like spinach and kale makes them ideal for usage in salads, smoothies, and even as a side dish to complement your favorite main meals. And let's not overlook the powerhouse that is broccoli, which, in addition to having a low glycemic index, is also rich in fiber and a variety of important elements.

In this chapter, we will go further into the world of fruits and vegetables, giving you with techniques to include them into your regular meals. These tactics will help you maintain a healthy diet and improve your overall well-being. In this lesson, we will examine a variety of delicious dishes and straightforward methods of preparation that may turn nutrient-dense foods into a delectable and reliable component of your diet.

As you read this chapter, keep in mind that a diet that is favorable to glucose is not about restriction; rather, it is about selecting choices that are both well-informed and delightful. Your home is complete with a refuge in the shape of your kitchen, and a change awaits you in the cupboards of your pantry. This is the beginning of your road toward stable blood sugar, and the way is lined with tastes, colors, and a world of possibilities in the kitchen.

Chapter 4

Protein, Fats, and Blood Sugar

As we continue on our quest to understand how to keep blood sugar under control, we have finally arrived at the most important aspect of a healthy diet: the dynamic relationship that exists between protein and fat. These dietary components, which are sometimes overlooked because of the emphasis placed on carbs, have equally important functions in maintaining stable blood glucose levels and fostering general health.

Protein's Role in Blood Sugar Control

Protein, which is known as the "building block of life," performs a wide variety of roles inside of our bodies. Not only does it help in the development and repair of tissues, but it also plays a function in controlling blood sugar, which is rather surprising but nevertheless quite important. How is it that it is able to do this?

When you eat meals that are high in protein, the proteins in those foods are broken down by your digestive system into their component amino acids. Amino acids are the basic building blocks of proteins. In contrast to the absorption of carbohydrates, the absorption of these amino acids into the circulation occurs at a more measured and consistent speed.

As a consequence of this, the slow release of amino acids has a moderate effect on the levels of sugar in the blood.

The splendor of this procedure resides in the fact that it is able to minimize the dramatic spikes and falls in blood sugar that are often linked with meals that are heavy in carbohydrates. It gives you a feeling of energy that lasts throughout the day, which may be very helpful for those who are trying to keep their blood glucose levels under control.

However, maintaining a healthy equilibrium is essential in all aspects of life. Even while protein may help stabilize blood sugar levels, eating too much of it might have the opposite effect. A condition known as gluconeogenesis, in which the body turns extra protein into glucose, may be brought on by eating an excessive amount of protein, particularly that which comes from animal sources. Therefore, it is vital to consume protein in a way that is considered as well as well-balanced.

Healthy Fats and Their Benefits

Let's shift our focus now to the realm of good fats, which is a topic that is sometimes misunderstood yet has incredible practical applications. We now understand that fats are not the nutritional monsters that they were originally thought to be, despite the fact that in the past they were unfairly demonized and given a bad name.

Avocados, nuts, seeds, and olive oil all include healthy fats, which may have a significant positive effect on a person's ability to regulate their blood sugar levels as well as their general state of health. They contribute significantly to the process of lowering the pace of digestion and absorption of carbs, which in turn helps to keep blood sugar levels steady.

Furthermore, the absorption of fat-soluble vitamins (A, D, E, and K) and other important nutrients is dependent on the presence of these fats. In addition to this, they induce feelings of satiety and fullness, which makes it more difficult to give in to the temptation of snacking on foods that mess with one's blood sugar levels.

You may further improve the glucose-friendly character of your meals by adding healthy fats to your diet. This will create a harmonic balance that will support your efforts to maintain stable blood sugar levels.

Achieving Balance: Proteins and Fats

After going over the separate functions that protein and healthy fats play in the regulation of blood sugar, the next step that makes sense is to find a balance between the two in the foods that you eat. Obtaining this equilibrium is not just dependent on scientific knowledge; rather, it requires the preparation of meals that are not only delectable but also beneficial to the achievement of one's own health objectives.

Finding the right ratio of carbs, proteins, and lipids is an art form. It involves awareness as well as a willingness to try out a variety of different combinations of foods in order to determine which ones work best for you. To help you started, here are some useful hints and suggestions:

Create Balanced Meals: Aim to include a source of lean protein (like chicken, fish, or tofu), healthy fats (such as avocados or nuts), and carbohydrates (preferably with a low glycemic index) in each meal.

Snack Wisely: If you're snacking between meals, choose options that combine protein and healthy fats. A handful of nuts with some veggies or a small serving of Greek yogurt with berries can be excellent choices.

Portion Control: Remember that fats are calorie-dense, so portion control is crucial. A little healthy fat can go a long way in enhancing the flavor and nutrition of your meals.

Experiment with Cooking Methods: Explore various cooking methods like grilling, roasting, or sautéing to bring out the best in your protein and fat sources.

A diet that strikes the right balance between carbs, proteins, and fats may result in more sustained energy, enhanced satiety, and better regulation of blood sugar levels. It is an essential component of the strategy that is presented in the Glucose Revolution book, and it gives you the opportunity to maintain your health and vigor in a manner that is both flexible and pleasant.

When you're trying to keep your blood sugar levels steady, it's crucial to remember that the foods you choose to eat are your secret weapon. Proteins and fats are going to be your friends on this trip, and if you can grasp the roles that they play and strike a balance between the two, you will give yourself even more ability to take charge of your health and wellbeing. Continue on this path of change with the knowledge that each mouthful we consume has the potential to get us closer to a life that is both healthier and more lively.

Chapter 5

Physical Activity and Blood Sugar

We sometimes find ourselves in a sedentary dance among the hectic rhythms of life, with our body languishing on the sofa or swaying softly in office chairs as we go about our daily routines. But what if we told you that inside the world of physical exercise lies a fundamental secret to regulating your blood sugar and, in consequence, your health? How would you react to such information? This mystery will be solved in the next section as we investigate the complex link that exists between exercise and the regulation of blood sugar levels.

Creating a Sustainable Workout Routine

Now, the issue that has to be asked is, "How can one sustainably integrate physical activity into their daily lives?" The goal is to choose things that you love doing, since this will enhance the probability that you will continue participating in them over the long term. Choose activities that get you excited to move your body, such as dancing, hiking, swimming, or lifting weights. This will help you stay motivated to move more.

Think about establishing objectives that are both precise and attainable. It's possible that they're connected to the length, the frequency, or the intensity. You may, for instance, set a goal to walk for a total of half an hour every single day or to do a certain amount of exercises each week. On your path to improved management of your blood sugar, these objectives will serve as important milestones.

It is essential to strike a personal equilibrium that serves your needs. A balanced exercise routine should include both aerobic activities, such as running or cycling, and strength training, which helps grow and maintain muscle mass. Because muscle tissue is so efficient at using glucose, increasing your muscle mass may help you become more sensitive to the effects of insulin.

Also, don't forget about yoga and other forms of relaxation and flexibility training like tai chi and yoga, which may help decrease stress, which is a prevalent factor that contributes to variations in blood sugar levels. Your entire health may be significantly improved by taking a comprehensive approach to physical training.

Tailoring Exercise to Your Glucose Goals

Exercising is not a one-size-fits-all approach, and the effect it has on a person's blood sugar levels might differ depending on the individual. It is crucial to understand how various forms of exercise influence your body in order to customize your workouts to the glycemic targets you have set for yourself.

Cardiovascular Exercise: Running, swimming, and cycling are all great ways to get some exercise and bring down your blood sugar levels. It is well known that they have an immediate effect on lowering blood sugar rises that occur after a meal. Include these workouts in your regimen if improving your insulin sensitivity and better managing your blood sugar is something you want to work toward.

Strength Training: Increasing the amount of muscle you have and keeping it at a healthy level are both excellent ways to speed up your metabolic rate and make your body more effective at regulating glucose levels. Even while the immediate effects on blood sugar management may not be as evident as they are with cardiovascular exercise, the long-term advantages could be rather large.

High-Intensity Interval Training (HIIT): Workouts using the HIIT method consist of strong bursts of activity followed by intervals of relatively light activity for recuperation. These exercises have the potential to bring about fast reductions in blood sugar levels as well as improvements in insulin sensitivity. They are effective in saving you time and may be a wonderful addition to your regular routine.

Mind-Body Exercises: Not only can practices like yoga and tai chi aid with flexibility and relieving tension, but they also have the potential to contribute to the control of blood sugar levels. Reducing stress is necessary because the chemicals produced in response to stress might promote high blood sugar levels.

Timing Matters: Think about when you should be doing your workout. Exercising before a meal may assist those who are prone to it get their post-meal blood sugar increases under control. Try out a few different timings and keep an eye on how your body reacts to each one.

Keep in mind that the immediate impacts of exercise are not as important as the long-term advantages as you begin your path toward improved blood sugar management via exercise. If you make physical activity a regular part of your life, you will discover that the advantages extend beyond simply your blood sugar levels and extend to your entire health, vigor, and sense of well-being.

Chapter 6

Monitoring and Managing Your Glucose

Welcome to the most important chapter of "The Glucose Revolution Method," which will help you unleash the method's full potential to revolutionize your life. This chapter will bridge the gap between information and action. In this chapter, we will discuss one of the most important aspects of your health journey:

monitoring and controlling your glucose levels.

The Importance of Regular Monitoring.

Imagine you had a map that will always lead you in the direction of achieving your best possible state of health. Maintaining a consistent monitoring schedule for your blood glucose levels is the compass you need. It is not just a routine; rather, it is your window into the dynamic world of the energy control in your body.

You may acquire significant insights into how your body reacts to various meals, activities, and stresses by checking your blood glucose on a daily basis. Because you now have this information, you have the ability to make educated choices regarding your food and lifestyle, so ensuring that you continue along the road of maintaining stable blood sugar levels.

However, monitoring involves more than just looking at data on a screen. It is a voyage of self-discovery as well as a process that brings you more in touch with your own body. It encourages attention and awareness, which lays the groundwork for a deep comprehension of the subtle dance that takes place between your decisions and your well-being.

Interpreting Your Glucose Readings

Your blood glucose measurements are not an exception to the rule that numbers always tell a narrative. In this part of the article, we will decipher the story that is concealed behind those numerals. What does the presence of spikes and dips imply? How does your body respond to the consumption of certain foods? Which patterns become more apparent as time passes?

We walk you through the process of interpretation and provide you the skills you need to understand what your blood glucose measurements are trying to tell you about their meaning. With this information at your disposal, you will be able to see patterns, pinpoint triggers, and predict how your body will react to a variety of scenarios.

Knowing how to read your glucose levels is not only about taking care of a problem; it's also about having complete control over your own physiology. It's about taking back control of your life and directing your health in the direction you want it to go.

Adjusting Your Diet and Lifestyle

It is time to take significant action now that you are armed with the insights acquired from monitoring and understanding the data. This section serves as your guide to making changes to your diet and lifestyle that will have a substantial impact.

Learn the ins and outs of putting up a customized diet that is low in glucose and caters to your specific requirements. Figure out how to make adjustments to your meal plans in order to keep a stable level of blood sugar throughout the day. Investigate the symbiotic link that exists between physical activity and the management of glucose, as well as the manner in which seemingly little alterations may lead to significant outcomes.

However, this is not a set-in-stone instruction manual; rather, it is an adaptable guide that follows the path of your adventure. We provide you the tools to make decisions that are in line with your tastes and the way you live your life, all while putting your wellbeing in the front.

Monitoring and controlling your glucose levels is not a chore in the quest of optimum health; rather, it is a process that is both dynamic and powerful. It's a voyage of self-discovery, a vow to yourself for a life filled with energy, and a dedication to learning about and taking care of your body.

Prepare yourself to take control of the situation, analyze the clues, and implement the changes that will move you farther down the road to a healthier and more energetic version of yourself. This is the beginning of your revolution against glucose.

Chapter 7

Beyond Diabetes: Glucose for Life

We are excited to see you reach this point in your Glucose Revolution adventure. In this chapter, we go beyond the confines of diabetes and reveal a road map to not just controlling glucose but also embracing a life that is brimming with energy. This is a life in which glucose is not a barrier but rather a partner on your journey to achieve maximum well-being.

Preventing Type 2 Diabetes

The risk of developing type 2 diabetes is significant in the contemporary medical environment. But you have nothing to worry about since knowledge is power. We are going to go on a journey of prevention, which will provide you with the insights and methods you need to strengthen your defenses against this common ailment that may often be avoided.

Learn the science underlying type 2 diabetes, discover the impact that genetics and lifestyle play in the disease, and find out how apparently insignificant decisions may create a barrier against the disease's development. We provide you the tools you need to rewrite your health narrative, from the potential of a Glucose-Friendly

Diet to the life-changing effects of engaging in regular physical activity.

Explore a variety of helpful hints, mouthwatering recipes, and improvements to your lifestyle that will not only reduce your risk of developing diabetes but will also improve your overall health. The goal of prevention should not be limited to only avoiding a diagnosis; rather, it should be to embrace a life that is full of vitality, resilience, and longevity.

Glucose Management in Special Situations

The trip that is life is filled with unexpected detours and turns, and there are moments when exceptional actions are required. under this part of the article, we will discuss the complex and delicate art of managing glucose levels under unusual circumstances. We provide individualized counsel to help you negotiate these issues without sacrificing your glucose objectives, whether it's because you're pregnant, under a lot of stress, sick, or have specific dietary demands.

Explore the complexities of controlling your blood sugar while pregnant, including the influence that stress has on your glucose levels, and devise a strategy that can be adapted to your specific conditions in order to get optimal results. This is not a cookie-cutter method; rather, it is a tailored guide to regulating your glucose levels within the rich tapestry of life.

Living a Glucose-Healthy Life

Beyond the area of preventive and exceptional situations lies the core of the Glucose Revolution, which is a way of life in which glucose is not a constraining force but rather a partner in your road to better health. We explore the practice of leading a life that is low in glucose, in which each decision we make leads to our continued health and happiness.

Discover the pleasure of living a healthy life while eating delectable meals that provide nourishment for both the body and the spirit. Learn the tricks of the mindfulness and stress management trade by gaining an awareness of how these components are intertwined with the process of glucose control. This is not simply about keeping track of statistics;

rather, it is about adopting a way of life that is congruent with the objectives you have set for your health.

As you go through this chapter, try to picture a life in which glucose is not a constraint but rather a factor that contributes to an exciting and satisfying lifestyle. Your Glucose Revolution is the key to unlocking the possibilities that exist beyond the realm of diabetes. the diabetic panorama of possibilities. You have reached the point in your trip toward a healthy life filled with pleasure and vigor where glucose will join you as a travel companion.

Conclusion

Taking Responsibility for Your Own Health. You have now arrived at the zenith of a life-altering adventure as you come to the end of The Glucose Revolution Method. This journey has taken you not only through the words contained in these pages, but also through the very fabric of your day-to-day existence. This chapter is not just a conclusion; rather, it is a fresh beginning, a call to action, and a celebration of the increased power over your health that you have achieved.

Embracing the Power Within

Throughout this book, you have dug into the complexities of blood glucose regulation, explored the science underlying the Glycemic Index, and improved your abilities in constructing a Glucose-Friendly Diet. In addition, you have gained an understanding of how the Glycemic Index was developed. You have mastered the skill of producing meals that are nourishing to both the body and the spirit by striking the proper balance between carbs, proteins, and fats. However, there is a power that resides beyond the information itself, and that power is the ability to make decisions that will feed your energy.

A Lifelong Journey

Taking charge of your health is not a one-time event; rather, it is a decision to commit to a journey that will last a lifetime. It's about beginning each day with a refreshed feeling of purpose, equipped with the awareness that your decisions have an impact on your overall health and happiness. This path will not be without its difficulties, but each difficulty represents a chance for personal development, education, and resiliency.

Celebrating Progress, Not Perfection

When it comes to one's health, the pursuit of perfection is not the aim; rather, progress is. Celebrate the minor triumphs, such as the days on which you decide to snack on something wholesome, the moments in which you choose to participate in physical exercise, and the times when you listen to your body. Recognize that health is a notion that encompasses the whole person, and that making healthy decisions helps to your total well-being.

Beyond the Book

The ideas presented in The Glucose Revolution Method are not limited to the pages that you are now reading. They are designed to be incorporated into your normal routine in some way. As you get to the end of this chapter, you should give some thought to the creation of a personal roadmap. This is a list of objectives and strategies that will help you stay on the route that leads to health and vitality. Your adventure does not come to a stop with the book; rather, it develops into a bespoke and environmentally responsible way of life.

Building a Resilient Mindset

The cultivation of a tough mental attitude is an essential component of overall health, alongside the maintenance of a healthy physical body. Embrace the difficulties, make the most of the opportunities to grow that the setbacks provide, and meet each new day with a feeling of wonder and compassion for yourself. Your frame of mind is a strong ally on your trip; it will shape the experiences you have and will influence the decisions you make.

Connecting with Your Why

As you think back on the information you've received and the adjustments you've made, connect with your "why." Why did you decide to go through with this trip? Whether it be to feel more energetic, avoid disease, or just live your best life, maintaining your objectives at the forefront of your mind will fuel your commitment.

Your Health, Your Revolution

As we get to the end of The Glucose Revolution Method, it is important to keep in mind that your health is your revolution. It's a never-ending cycle of getting to know oneself better, taking care of oneself, and giving oneself more agency. Your perseverance and determination are on display in the fact that you are now in complete command of your health. It's a celebration of the one-of-a-kind and very strong person that you are.

As you flip the last page, keep in mind that the ideas presented in this book are more than simply information; they are instruments that may be used to fashion a life that is rich in energy, wellbeing, and satisfaction. The Glucose Revolution is now yours to experience, to enjoy, and to spread with others. I pray that your travels are spectacular and that the immense strength that is inside you is reflected in the state of your health.